In
Control!

In Control!

Everything You Need to Know About Worry-Free, Joyful Sex

MADELINE Y. SUTTON, MD, MPH

publish
yⓕur gift

IN CONTROL!
Copyright © 2021 Madeline Y. Sutton
All rights reserved.

Published by Publish Your Gift®
An imprint of Purposely Created Publishing Group, LLC

Printed in the United States of America

ISBN: 978-1-64484-369-7 (print)
ISBN: 978-1-64484-370-3 (ebook)

Special discounts are available on bulk quantity purchases by book clubs, associations and special interest groups. For details email: sales@publishyourgift.com or call (888) 949-6228.
For information log on to www.PublishYourGift.com

"Caring for myself is not self-indulgence, it is self-preservation, and that is an act of political warfare."

—Audre Lorde

For my father and mother,
who instilled pride and resilience in me and who set me
on a path to realize as many of my dreams as possible.

For my sons, Azia, Mehki, and Mason,
who are the wind beneath my wings and who inspire me to
reach higher every day. Parenting them is my ultimate joy.

TABLE OF CONTENTS

FOREWORD

From our current positions as national leaders in medicine and advocacy, Madeline and I can look back to 30 years ago when we met. We were classmates at Columbia Medical School in New York City (College of Physicians and Surgeons), a new place to me but home for Madeline. We became fast friends; we laughed a lot and didn't take ourselves too seriously. But we were serious about our work in that demanding time of growth and maturation. We also bonded quickly in our passion for women's health and desire to do some good. We share a deep appreciation for how feminist scholars—especially Audre Lorde—inform our medical practice. It's easy to see how we both ended up choosing obstetrics and gynecology for our physician career paths. We love helping women!

I reconnected with Dr. Sutton years later through our advocacy work with Physicians for Reproductive Health. Madeline is a perfect advocate for reproductive justice; she made deep inroads in sexual health and HIV prevention through her research at the Centers for Disease Control and Prevention (CDC), always informed by on-the-ground, hands-on medicine. Her scientific work rippled outward, informing policy to fight harmful legislation. She is my favorite kind of doctor; she sees the whole picture and takes on the challenge to make things right.

We're at another crossroads in the evolution of women's health in the United States with a new Supreme Court Justice (Barrett); no doubt, challenges lay ahead. In times of uncertainty, this book is key for people who are interested in birth control and need to know more. First, Dr. Sutton takes a scientific and user-friendly look at the complex and racialized history of birth control in the United States. Then, she discusses options currently available and how fuller utilization allows us to live a reality in which we can decide and if and when to be pregnant. Birth control allows people reproductive control, and that control allows freedom within their sexual lives.

What I know for sure is that Dr. Sutton and I are in this for the long run. We will help women get what they need. You will undoubtedly enjoy this book by my friend, colleague, fellow New Yorker, and women's health warrior, Dr. Madeline Sutton; she will help you get what YOU need.

Anne R. Davis, MD, MPH
Director, Family Planning Fellowship, Columbia University Department of Obstetrics and Gynecology
Past Board Member and Consulting Medical Director, Physicians for Reproductive Health
Professor, Columbia University Irving Medical Center, Department of Obstetrics and Gynecology

INTRODUCTION

For many women, freedom is directly tied to their reproductive choices and options, yet many women don't feel fully informed about those options and which ones are safest and most effective for them. I wrote this book to honor as many women as possible by helping them get in control and have more freedom, as much freedom as possible. Once women are empowered with their knowledge of choices, they alone control their bodies, their reproductive choices, and ultimately their sexuality and sexual pleasure. I've watched so many patients, friends, and colleagues, women who are often so busy moving around and putting others' needs ahead of their own, forget about what they themselves need, what brings them joy, and what control looks like for them. I know because I've been there.

I was born and raised in New York City. Harlem is my home; it is there that I met and was nourished by an extended village of people who loved and supported me. I wanted to be a doctor starting at age eight when I had my ears pierced at a Black male pediatrician's office in Harlem; that feeling was reaffirmed at age thirteen when a young surgical resident at Columbia-Presbyterian Hospital (who did my appendectomy) was kind enough to show me my appendix after it was removed. My mom and dad supported me however they could; we had a steep learning curve as I was their oldest child and the first in the family to attend college. I graduated from the Bronx High School of Science. I fell in love with Georgetown University the first time I visited the campus after being accepted to attend. I finished both Columbia University College of Physicians and Surgeons and the Mailman School of Public Health in four years with my joint MD, MPH degrees. After completing my OB/GYN residency, I joined the Centers for Disease Control and Prevention, served as a Commissioned Corps Officer of the United States Public Health Service for twenty-one and a half years, and authored and co-authored a book and more than 150 peer-reviewed scientific articles about sexual health and women's health. I've been a board-certified OB/GYN for over twenty years. I also maintained a clinical practice through a community health center and Morehouse School of Medicine, providing care for a diverse group of women and helping educate them regarding their obstetric and gynecologic concerns, birth control options, and overall health.

While all this was happening, I got married, gave birth to my three beautiful sons, held down several jobs, attended my sons' sporting events, and covered household and educational expenses for our sons. I was holding it all down, but I was also exhausted. I didn't have enough hours in the day. I started to feel like I needed more help as a busy, working mom. Who else can identify with that? Like many of you, I was taking care of my family and trying to maintain my health and my sexy. One day, after a really intense several months of work, I hit rock bottom. I had to stop because the reality was I was burning myself out, and I couldn't do it all. I sought counseling, tried to fix the things that were wrong, and ultimately, I started to prioritize me. What could I control? How could I feel my freedom? How could I maintain my health and my sexy? I knew that I couldn't continue in the same way.

So, I shifted. I took control of my life. As I became more confident, I found healing moments in self-care, in more deliberate mom-son time, in more traveling, in sister-friend time, and in freedom. I started my road to healing and rearranged some things and did things differently. It was not easy, but it was necessary, and I not only survived, I thrived.

I had more freedom, and I formulated what it would look like to help other women, whether partnered or not, access more freedom. And that became my purpose because freedom looks different for every woman, although some parts of women's struggles are similar. And like the famous poet Audre Lorde said, "I am not free while any woman is unfree, even when her shackles are different from my own." So, I do this work because I am passionate about helping every woman reach her own freedom. And I am passionate about helping as many women as possible be in control.

I wrote this book in three parts: Part One provides historical context for birth control in the US; it's not a pretty history, so I address it straight on. Part Two updates women on what is currently available as birth control options for women in the US. Part Three starts the discussion of what control and freedom might look like for you. Each part opens with a quote from a powerful woman, and each quote is about women and control. In each chapter, I start with condensed quotes of things said to me by many patients over the years; they are not quotes specific to one person. I start that way, so that each person knows that no question or comment is "silly" or "stupid." I've heard it all, and it's important to talk about the questions and comments that folks have in order to dispel the myths head-on. I also included some fast facts at the start of every chapter for those who appreciate getting information in nuggets. I've written this book to be user-friendly with some science and data thrown in, so that you have what you need to make informed decisions about your worry-free, joyful sex lives. So, with all of that said, let's go get in control.

PART I.

HISTORICAL CONTEXT

"Contraceptive protection is something every woman must have access to, to control her own destiny."

—Ruth Bader Ginsberg

CHAPTER 1.
Real Talk: A Brief History of Birth Control in the United States, Impact on Women of Color, and Where We Are Today

FAST FACTS:

- History isn't always pretty, but knowledge is always power.

- Conversations about birth control today should always feel voluntary and in support of your personal and/or professional goals for yourself.

There is joy and power in knowing and controlling one's own body. Throughout history and even in 2021, in many parts of the world, what happens to women's bodies has often been controlled by others. Controlling women's ability to bear children and controlling what women feel or don't feel during sex has been part of the global struggle since the beginning of time. And we've come a long way since then. In many parts of the world, women have gained full equality, and they alone are in control of their bodies, their lifestyles, their career paths (inside of or outside of the home), their families, their choices, and their sexuality. In other places in the world, including the United States, women continue to fight for control and equality in everything from birth control to how they are paid to do the same jobs as men to how they manage their sexual freedom.

Knowledge about and access to birth control or contraception is key for many women because it allows them to plan for many major events in their lives. When and whether to have children has helped women navigate many aspects of their lives, including the ability to live as freely as possible on their own terms, short-term and long-term educational and employment goals, personal development goals, travel desires, and family planning goals. So, understandably, women have been experimenting with ways to manage their fertility for centuries.

Historically in the US, there are many documented reports of women cleverly using various methods as contraception. It is documented that as early as 1619 through the 1800s, Black/African American women relied on herbal methods from African folklore in an effort to resist coerced reproduction by white men who had enslaved them. Native American women used blue cohosh and other substances to result in uterine contractions or a spermicidal effect to prevent pregnancies. In the 1870s, when an assortment of devices such as condoms, sponges, and syringes became available mostly for white women in America, the Comstock Law was quickly implemented by Congress. The Comstock Law made it illegal for contraceptives to move across state lines through the US Postal Service. At this time in the 1870s, the US was the only western nation to criminalize birth control.

By 1914, Margaret Sanger, the founder of what is today known as Planned Parenthood Federation of America, was credited with coining the term "birth control," and she began her efforts to educate women in the US and abroad about their contraceptive options. Although Sanger's efforts evolved to appeal to all women regardless of race and ethnicity, her initial efforts were aligned with unethical eugenic activities that were designed to decrease pregnancies among women of color in the early 1900s. The practice of eugenics or "the study of how to arrange reproduction within a human population to increase the occurrence of heritable characteristics regarded as desirable" was developed largely by Sir Francis Galton as a method of "improving" the human race. Eugenics was discredited as unscientific and racially biased during the twentieth century, especially after the adoption of its doctrines by the Nazis to justify their treatment of Jews, disabled people, and other minority groups. In the US, eugenics against Black/African American women, Hispanic women/Latinas, and Native American women continued through the 1970s through unethical and illegal sterilizations performed by members of the medical establishment. Even initial studies on birth control pills, which were first developed in the 1960s, included large numbers of women in Puerto Rico, who were not only unethically enrolled in many cases but who also suffered a disproportionate number of deaths due to side effects from a birth control pill that had significantly higher doses of hormones than birth control pills available in 2021. Sadly, even as recently as 2020, there were reports of Spanish-speaking women in the state of Georgia, being victimized by a medical establishment that removed their uteruses (did hysterectomies) without their consent. (For those who may be interested in learning more about the history of birth control, please visit the website for Our Bodies Ourselves: https://www.ourbodiesourselves.org/ book-excerpts/health-article/a-brief-history-of-birth-control/). This is all-important history to understand as we consider the modern-day conversations about birth control.

This historical context underscores why some Black and brown women and men, even today, question the intent of birth control options and remain untrusting of some medical personnel as it relates to this topic. The goal of this book is to inform readers regarding available birth control science in the most transparent way possible, so that all women, especially women of color, can be even more empowered as they make decisions and take control of their contraceptive choices (1). For many women, especially women of color, access to contraceptives intersects with the three primary principles of "reproductive justice:" 1) the right to not have a child, 2) the right to have a child, and 3) the right to parent children in safe and healthy environments (2). These principles underscore that the 99 percent of women in America who report using birth control at some point in their lives should always have contraceptive counseling that is patient-centered, informative, and evidence-based, always asking women what matters to them most, and always respecting their preferences. This is especially important for the almost 20 million reproductive age women (ages eleven to fifty-one years who have regular menstrual cycles) who lack private insurance or self-pay access or who live in areas that don't have health centers which offer all contraceptive options (3).

Today, there are many safe and effective birth control options available for women of all races and ethnicities, and they have been rigorously and ethically studied in many groups of women who gave consent and volunteered to participate. As Queen-Mother Maya Angelou used to say, "When you know better, you do better." While we are doing better regarding safe and effective contraceptives for women (and other non-binary, gendered persons who may be able to become pregnant), we cannot let our guard down. It remains important that women be informed about and can access the full range of safe, available birth control that they need, especially as we continue to navigate through new and ongoing federal and local legal challenges that seek to chip away at these fundamental reproductive rights for women. Decreased access to birth control contributes to the unintended pregnancy rate in the US, which hovers around 50 percent. By strengthening access to birth control, we can help decrease the unintended pregnancy rate (which also contributes to subsequent abortions) that has been part of the American reproductive health dialogue for decades. Women who use contraception consistently and correctly account for only 5 percent of unintended pregnancies.

Today's contraceptive options include birth control pills, intrauterine devices (IUDs), subdermal implants, injections, vaginal rings, patches, condoms, and emergency contraceptives when all else fails. Development of new birth control options is an ongoing process. One of the things that brings me the most joy as a board-certified OB/GYN is helping to educate women of all ages and from all walks of life about what options are available to them and answering their questions based on their specific scenarios and without judgment. Many women describe feeling more control and freedom when they decide whether or not and when they might want to have children; so, birth control use can be extremely liberating.

There is no one-size-fits-all (or most) when it comes to birth control. In this book, we'll review each birth control method by starting with real-talk questions and quotes from women, up-to-date scientific information, and resources for how you can access what you need. During my twenty plus years of taking care of women as patients, I've heard many questions and concerns, and so the quotes you see at the start of each chapter are intended to provide real-life context. I always reassure my patients that there is no such thing as a silly question, only questions that we are sometimes too shy or too nervous to ask. By including questions in this way, I want to help you feel empowered to seek answers to all of your questions, especially as they relate to birth control and worry-free, joyful sex. I also included a few fast facts at the start of each chapter to try to address a few frequently asked questions or share a few pearls I've picked up along my journey. With the information in this book, you are in control. You decide what's right for you. You get to move closer to the freedom that you desire and deserve. So, let's get started.

PART II.

WHAT BIRTH CONTROL OPTIONS ARE CURRENTLY AVAILABLE TO YOU?

"Freeing yourself was one thing, claiming ownership of that freed self was another."

—Toni Morrison

CHAPTER 2.

"That pill had me spotting, and I kept forgetting to take it, so I just stopped taking it."

The Pill

FAST FACTS:

- There are over 100 birth control brands with varying amounts of hormones available in the US. If one brand or type doesn't work, talk with your clinician about trying an alternative option.

- Some irregular spotting or bleeding will stop after the first two to three months of use.

- Many times, changing the type of pill or the hormone component can decrease or stop any prolonged bleeding.

Indeed, many of my patients have shared with me these exact concerns about spotting or forgetting their pills during these past two decades. In my twenties and thirties, I also had challenges with trying to remember to take the pill every day! Some days, I'd be in the middle of doing something and stop dead in my tracks trying to remember if I had taken a pill for that day, and more importantly, trying to recall if I had the pill pack with me, so I could check. Sometimes, remembering was as simple as trying to carry the same purse with the package in there or remembering to take the package out of the pocket of the jeans I had on the day before. My life was often too hectic to be as efficient as I needed to be to successfully take the pill preferably at the same time every day.

Still, the birth control pill ("The Pill") is the most commonly used reversible contraceptive option in the United States. It was used by an estimated 10.2 million sexually active women who were age fifteen to forty-nine-years-old or 14 percent of women who were using contraception, as of 2019. When used perfectly, the pill can be 99 percent effective. But we are human, naturally imperfect, often juggling multiple tasks and sometimes taking a pill late or perhaps forgetting to take it altogether for a day or two or three. So, with typical human use, the pill is 91 percent effective. That means that for every 100 women taking the pill for birth control, nine of them will get pregnant, and ninety-one of them won't get pregnant. As with each option, you have to decide what odds of failure and effectiveness will work best for you based on your day-to-day realities. I've known many patients who enjoy taking their daily birth control pill and have no problems at all; many use physical reminders by placing their pill packs near their toothbrush or make taking it a part of any routine that they tend to do at the same time every day. Also, these days, electronic reminders are available through phone apps.

There are several reasons for the popularity of the pill. First, we've had it available for contraceptive use in the US for the longest period of time compared with other options. When the Food and Drug Administration approved the first-ever birth control option in the US in the 1960s, it was the pill. Second, the pill immediately gave women who could access it more freedom to choose the timing of their pregnancies, more flexibility to pursue other educational and work ambitions, more opportunities to have sex without the worry of an unintended pregnancy, and a greater sense of owning their expanded freedoms. Third, with the modern-day formulations which have less hormones in them, there are fewer side effects, so birth control pills are more easily tolerated by women. Fourth, the pill can be easily stopped allowing for a shorter return to fertility when/if someone decides they are ready to start trying to have a baby. Fifth, in most cases, the cost of the pill is low, sometimes as low as $8-$10 per monthly package or with no co-pays at all with some insurance plans.

There are also many non-contraceptive benefits to the birth control pill. For many patients who have heavy bleeding or lots of pain during their menses, the pill regulates bleeding by producing a predictable cycle of bleeding. It also reduces menstrual-related pain. Using the pill can also reduce symptoms of some medical conditions such as endometriosis, migraines, endometrial cancer, and ovarian cancer. Because the pill works by suppressing ovulation (stopping the ovaries from releasing an egg), it also helps decrease premenstrual syndrome symptoms, helps shrink some ovarian cysts, and decreases fibrocystic breast changes. For pills that have both estrogen and progesterone components, the estrogen part can help improve acne, decrease excess hair growth in women, decrease perimenopausal symptoms, including hot flashes, and strengthen bones among some older, menopausal women.

For some women who might smoke cigarettes or have hypertension (high blood pressure), there are risks involved with taking the combination (two-hormone) pill, including deep venous thromboses (or blood clots in the legs), a stroke or a myocardial infarction (heart attack). For these patients, combination pills are not recommended; I always counsel these patients regarding either a progesterone-only method, or even better, non-hormonal options for birth control. Decades of data have shown us that the risk is too high in these patients. Other medical conditions that would negate the use of combination birth control pills include: having a current deep venous thrombosis (DVT, or clot in the leg) or history of a DVT, coronary artery disease, diabetes mellitus with severe vascular disease, migraine headaches with aura, prolonged immobilization, current breast cancer, liver disease, lupus with antiphospholipid antibodies, and being less than twenty-one days postpartum (after delivering a baby).

So, what does it mean when we describe combination or two-hormone pills and progestin-only or one hormone pills? The main birth control options on the market are either combination (includes both estrogen and progestin) and progestin-only pills. They all work by preventing ovulation or the release of eggs from the ovaries. Therefore, they prevent fertilization by preventing any sperm that enters the vagina, uterus, or fallopian tube from having an egg to merge with to create an embryo. There are many different formulations for combination birth control pills. (Please go to Appendix 1 to see the different types of formulations that are possible for birth control pills; there are currently > 200 types of pills on the market.) Remember, if the pill you are taking is not working for you, talk with your doctor, nurse practitioner, or midwife about trying an alternative type of pill or a different form of contraception based on your needs. Pills differ based on the types of progestin components and also amounts of estrogen, and women often will be prescribed one formulation or another based on a desired benefit in addition to the contraceptive component. For example, some combination pills have the added benefit of decreasing acne in teenage and young adult women who might desire that additional benefit.

Progestin-only pills contain no estrogen and can be safe for women who are unable to take combination birth control pills. These progestin-only pills are most effective if they are taken at the same time every day or at least within three hours of that time. The most common complaint about the progestin-only pills is irregular bleeding or spotting that may happen in between a woman's cycle and disrupt her quality of life. Irregular bleeding or frequent spotting is a very common reason why women stop taking this type of pill and opt for a different type of contraception. Remember, with the pill and other forms of birth control, there's no protection against sexually transmitted infections (STIs), so it's important to remember to use a condom for protection and for more worry-free sex. Another approach that works for some sexually active people who use a non-barrier method of birth control is to be screened for most STIs, including Human Immunodeficiency Virus (HIV), together with their partner(s), whenever there is a new partner. The people who choose this path are often exploring ways to be sexually active in a fun and safe way without always using a condom. If you choose this approach, be sure to discuss it with your clinician, so that you are as informed as possible about risks and options.

There are also pills that are for extended use; women who take these prefer the continuous aspect and fewer numbers of menstrual cycles every year. For example, Seasonique® birth control pills are taken for ninety-one consecutive days to suppress a woman's menstrual cycle, so that she only has her menses four times per year. Like pills that allow monthly cycles, continuous cycle birth control pills prevent the ovaries from releasing an egg and thicken the mucous, so that sperm is less likely to reach an egg. Additional non-contraceptive benefits with these continuous-cycle birth control pills include decreased acne, decreased risk of ovarian cysts, and regulation of menstrual cycles.

The reality is that forgetting to take a birth control pill happens more frequently than you may think. Here are some things to keep in mind if you happen to forget to take your combination hormone pill for one or two or more days. If you miss one pill, take it as soon as you remember. If you miss two days of taking pills consecutively, take two as soon as you remember and two the next day also. If you've missed three pills in a row, you're at risk of getting pregnant if you've had sex during those three days. Talk with your provider to see if emergency contraception might be a good idea. As you finish out that pack of pills for the month, you may have some spotting, and you should use a back-up method for the next month to be sure. If you missed pills for four to five days, you may get your period; restart your pills after you've been off of them for five days. Now, if the pills you missed are during week four of the pack and only involve non-hormonal reminder pills, you will likely get your regular period and be okay to start your next pill pack as scheduled. When only reminder pills are missed, no back-up birth control is needed. As you can see, this can all get pretty complicated; always give a call to your healthcare provider if you have missed some pills and have any questions or concerns about what to do next.

As you can see, depending on what's going on in one's world, remembering to take a pill at the same time every day to optimize the effectiveness for pregnancy prevention can get a little overwhelming for some. For some women, I counsel them to incorporate the pill into their nighttime or after dinner routine; this is especially helpful for women who might report mild nausea when they take the pill. Taking the pill at night always helps you sleep through any nausea. Of course, if that side effect continues after two to three months on the pill, check with your clinician about whether an alternative pill might be better for you. There are too many birth control pill options on the market to not explore when you have an undesirable side effect.

CHAPTER 3.

"My friend told me that the IUD would make me sterile; is that true? Besides, my man said he could feel the string when we have sex. Is there anything else that will give me ten years of worry-free sex if I take this out?"

Intrauterine Devices (IUDs)

FAST FACTS:

- IUDs are extremely effective and safe for long-term birth control and can be safely in place for between three to twelve years.

- Modern-day IUDs are not the ones from the 1970s; today's IUDs are safe and do not cause pelvic infections or sterility.

- If someone has a seven-year-old IUD and changes their mind and wants their IUD removed at the one, two, or three-year mark, they can have it removed without question. It is always a woman's right to change her mind regarding her chosen birth control method.

- Sometimes, a male sex partner will say they feel the string during sex.

Intrauterine devices (IUDs) are in the category of contraceptives known as long-acting reversible contraception or LARCs. IUDs are small, plastic devices that are inserted into the uterus by medical providers to prevent pregnancy. During the 1970s, IUDs fell out of favor for many years due to the history of the Dalkon Shield IUD; this IUD was associated with an increased risk of pelvic infections and infected miscarriages and was removed from the market. So, for many years after that, women were not interested in IUDs due to concerns regarding safety and yes, even reports of sterility with the older versions of IUDs. However, concerns about infections and sterility are not true with modern-day IUDs. In 1984, new, safer versions of IUDs were made available, and since that time, IUDs have become increasingly popular. As of 2019, an estimated 9.1 million women age fifteen to forty-nine in the US were using an IUD for birth control or about 10 percent of sexually active women who were using birth control.

There are a few reasons for the popularity of IUDs; they are about 99.2 percent effective at preventing pregnancy. In other words, out of 100 persons who use an IUD, an estimated one person will get pregnant, and ninety-nine will not get pregnant. Another big reason for the popularity of the IUD is that once its placement is confirmed in the uterus, most women don't have to think about it for between three to twelve years! Talk about freedom. After the birth of my third child, I had an IUD placed at my postpartum visit that was able to stay for twelve years, and there was a peace of mind during that time that could not be replaced. That's what many of my patients who choose an IUD are most excited about…the ability to have a device in place that they know is highly effective against an unplanned pregnancy that they don't have to think about every day.

IUDs are also very cost-effective, especially when covered by insurance without co-pays. When not covered by insurance, the upfront costs for women can range from $500 to $1300 for the device, plus separate costs for insertion by a clinician, so this starting price point can definitely be a barrier for many. However, if you consider the fact that it can be in place for twelve years, compared with the monthly costs of the pill (if co-pays are charged) or Depo-Provera costs every three months, those costs add up over time and are likely higher after twelve years of use than the cost of one IUD in place for twelve years. One of the positive things about the Affordable Health Care Act (ACA) when it was signed into law in 2010 is that it provided for coverage of all FDA-approved contraceptive methods for women without co-pays. Since 2010, multiple legal challenges to the ACA have led to some employers not being willing to support IUDs for their employees if that was their selected method of birth control. Unfortunately, this legal shift has led to co-pays and high costs being a barrier for many people who may seek certain types of birth control, especially IUDs.

IUDs work by preventing the sperm and the egg from meeting, so that fertilization does not happen. They also work by thickening the cervical mucous, inhibiting sperm motility and function, and thinning the endometrium. Certain types of IUDs can also be used to decrease painful and heavy menstrual blood flow and reduce the risk of endometrial cancer.

IUDs also are shown to have high user satisfaction and rapid reversibility, so that someone can quickly return to fertility (three to six months) after the IUD is removed. Increasingly, IUD placement is done right after the end of a pregnancy or in the delivery room right after the baby and placenta have been delivered. In these situations, the string may be kept a little longer, so that it can be trimmed if needed at the six-week postpartum visit after the uterus has returned to normal size. As we learn more about the safety of self-removal, some women are asking that the IUD string be kept a little longer in case they need to or choose to reach into their vaginas and pull on the string to remove the IUD themselves. Please keep in mind that choosing to keep the IUD string longer could lead to a male sex partner saying that he feels the string during sex. Some men describe feeling "poked by the string." While that is not a common complaint, your clinician can certainly trim the IUD string to make it shorter when you request it in an effort to decrease any discomfort during sexual intercourse.

There are two categories of IUDs available: 1) non-hormonal, copper IUDs, and 2) hormonal, progestin-only IUDs. There is only one non-hormonal IUD available in the US, and that is the Copper T IUD also known as ParaGard˙. Because it has no hormones, it works great with women who have medical conditions like chronic hypertension that prevent the use of hormonal contraceptives. Although the FDA has approved the copper IUD for ten years, several studies have shown that it can safely remain in place and be effective for as many as twelve years. The copper IUD is ideal for someone who is certain about wanting a long-term birth control option, whether or not they've already had children. The copper IUD is the only contraceptive that allows for ten plus years of worry-free sex, unless someone gets their tubes tied. Importantly, the copper IUD is also very effective for emergency contraception, with a failure rate between zero and 0.09 percent. Newer data shows zero pregnancies when placed in the uterus between six and fourteen days after unprotected sex with a negative pregnancy test.

For the category of hormonal, progestin IUDs, there are currently four available in the US. Mirena˚ can be in place for up to seven years for contraception and can also be used separately to treat heavy menstrual bleeding and painful periods. Liletta˚ can also be in place up to seven years and was designed to be available for a low cost and available at public health clinics; ideally, this IUD can be available with less financial barriers. Kyleena˚ and Skyla˚ can be safely in place for up to five years and three years, respectively. Skyla˚ and Kyleena˚ are both smaller IUDs with lower hormone levels than Mirena˚ and Liletta˚. Although all have been safely used in women who have never had children, only Skyla˚ and Kyleena˚ are FDA-approved for use in women who have never had children. Importantly, any IUD can be removed before its maximum number of years; just let your clinician know if you change your mind and would like to take it out.

The main side effects with IUDs include changes in menstrual patterns, especially during the first few months after insertion. Usually any irregular bleeding resolves within three to four months after insertion. Rarely, an IUD can slip further up into a uterus that enlarges, making it difficult to find the string. In these cases, the IUD can still be removed, although it may have to be done outside of the doctor's office at the hospital. There are few contraindications to using an IUD, but they include someone who is already pregnant, someone who has an ongoing pelvic infection or other acute abnormality of the uterus, including types of fibroids that distort the cavity inside of the uterus, and someone who has a malignancy in the uterus, cervix or breast cancer (copper IUD can be used in someone who has had breast cancer, but not the hormonal IUD).

Things that should make you immediately call your clinician: 1) you suddenly cannot locate the string, in which case an ultrasound will be needed. (Many times an ultrasound will show that the IUD is still in place, just the string has moved higher into the cervix or uterus), 2) symptoms of pregnancy or infection, 3) sudden, unexplained pelvic pain, or 4) excessive and new onset heavy bleeding. Also, with about one to six out of 1000 persons, an IUD may cause a small hole in the uterus (perforation) and require same-day surgical removal. Most of these IUD issues are quickly resolved and do not cause long-term harm.

CHAPTER 4.

"Some of my friends have that plastic stick that goes in your arm. What's that about?"

Contraceptive Implants

FAST FACTS:

- The implant can be placed in less than ten minutes in an office or other private setting.

- The implant is placed discreetly in your upper arm. It can be there with or without a sex partner's awareness for those who need discretion.

- It can safely be in place for three to five years for pregnancy prevention.

That plastic stick is Nexplanon˙! Like the IUD, it is a long-acting reversible contraceptive or LARC. Nexplanon˙ is the only contraceptive implant currently available in the US. It is a narrow (0.2 mm), flexible rod, about 4 cm in length that is placed in the upper arm immediately beneath the skin. As of 2019, an estimated 2.9 million women or 4 percent of women who use birth control in the US had Nexplanon˙ as their contraceptive method. Nexplanon˙ is 99.95 percent effective as a birth control option; less than one person out of 100 will have a pregnancy when it is placed correctly. Nexplanon˙ is the only birth control method where effectiveness in typical everyday use is the same as perfect use. Placement must be done by a healthcare provider with local numbing medicine in an office setting; the same is required for removal. Both placement and removal can take as little as five to ten minutes. Although FDA has approved Nexplanon˚ for up to three years of use, several research studies show that it is safe and still prevents pregnancy for up to two additional years. So, it can be removed after five years of use or earlier, and if the person desires, it can be immediately replaced with a new device at the end of three to five full years of use. The ability to get pregnant can return as soon as the first week after removal.

Nexplanon˚ contains progestin hormones and works by preventing ovulation and by thickening the cervical mucous (mucous at the mouth of the womb) and thereby preventing sperm from penetrating. When the sperm can't get through, it can't meet an egg and cause fertilization. Benefits of the implant include that women can use it privately, with or without the knowledge of her partner; many women seek birth control that they can use discreetly without letting anyone know. One of the other great benefits of Nexplanon˚ is that it is effective among women of all weights and body mass indexes (BMIs). In this way, it differs from some other options, like the pill or vaginal ring that sometimes show evidence of less hormone in the system of women who are overweight or obese.

The main side effect of the implant is abnormal and unpredictable bleeding during the first few months after placement. During pre-placement counseling, informing patients about the irregular bleeding is the topic on which I spend the most time. It's a vital part of managing expectations. For patients who request removal of the implant before the three-year mark, it is most often due to dissatisfaction with the unpredictable bleeding. This is understandable because abnormal bleeding can disrupt the quality of life if it is really heavy or prolonged. Helping women navigate through this side effect increases the chance that they will try to maintain the implant until this side effect subsides. Many of my patients who reach five to six months of use often describe lighter and shorter periods, and sometimes their periods stop altogether. Other reported side effects with the implant include headaches, weight gain, acne, breast pain, depression, and abdominal pain, but these are all reported much less frequently than irregular menses.

The medical condition for which Nexplanon˙ can absolutely not be used is current or recent breast cancer (in the past five years). A malignant liver tumor is also a situation in which an implant should be used with caution.

The professional organization of board-certified obstetricians and gynecologists (ACOG or the American College of Obstetricians and Gynecologists) has recommended LARCs as options that should be discussed with women and adolescents seeking first-line contraception if appropriate based on her wants, needs, and risk factors. Studies have shown that LARCs are twenty times more effective at preventing an untimely pregnancy compared with birth control pills, the vaginal ring, and the patch. Both ACOG and the American Academy of Pediatrics (AAP) agree that LARCs are safe for all women regardless of age or whether or not they have given birth. This is important because years ago the mindset was that teenagers and/or someone who had not yet delivered a baby were not good candidates for LARCs. Research has shown that's not true. I have patients from adolescents to mature in age who have successfully had IUDs placed, especially now with some smaller-sized options, and done very well with them in place.

LARCs are also great because they reduce user error. They are inserted by trained clinicians for long-term placement and use, so the need to remember a daily, weekly, or monthly method is removed; this contributes to their high user satisfaction rates. So, depending on where you are in your contraceptive journey, LARCs are a great option for all of us to be aware of in case they are the method we choose to help move toward greater control and freedom.

CHAPTER 5.

"My cousin said she gained thirty pounds on that birth control shot, Doc. You think that was because of the medicine?"

The Shot, Depo-Provera®

FAST FACTS:

- The most common side effects of Depo-Provera® are irregular bleeding, spotting in between periods, and weight gain. These usually all resolve within the first year of use. If they don't resolve, these are all common reasons for women discontinuing the shot.

- Many women like the fact that they stop having a period altogether after they've been on the shot for a full year.

- Studies have shown that Depo-Provera® can be linked to weight gain for some women. If that happens with you, talk with your doctor about trying a different method and some ways to lose any weight gained while on Depo-Provera®.

Depo-Provera® or "the shot" is a highly safe and effective form of birth control. With typical use, it prevents 94 percent of pregnancies, so out of 100 women, six will experience an unintended pregnancy in the first year of use. Although it was used by 2.3 million women in the US in 2019, it is also the method that patients have the most questions about when it comes to irregular bleeding and weight gain. Many ladies will report that a good friend or family member gained weight on the shot. There was a study several years ago that showed that 25 percent of women gained weight (5 percent of their body weight) during the first three to six months of use; for those women, stopping the shot and switching to a non-hormonal method helped them take the weight off. But for 75 percent of women, there is no weight gain when they are on the shot.

So, what exactly is Depo-Provera®? Depo-Provera is a birth control method that uses progestin to prevent pregnancy by suppressing ovulation and is administered as an injection every twelve weeks. Although it's normally given in an office setting by a healthcare provider, if the person is comfortable, many opt to pick it up at the pharmacy and give it to themselves at home. Increasingly, exploring this option became more important during the recent COVID-19 public health emergency when many people were unable to access their doctors' offices to receive their injections. Many people gave themselves the injections at home. Also, the Depo-SubQ Provera increased in popularity as an option because it is given right under the skin (not as deep as the regular Depo shot) into one's stomach or upper thigh area every twelve to fourteen weeks.

One of the benefits that many women enjoy most when they are on Depo is that most have lighter and less painful periods after the initial months of irregular bleeding. For some women who use the shot consistently for more than twelve months, their menstrual cycles may stop altogether, which many women enjoy as a side effect. Some women ask me if it's safe to not have a period. "Is my womb holding on to that blood? Doesn't it need to come out of my body somehow?" The good news is that it's completely safe. When you are on Depo-Provera`, your ovaries are resting, so the lining of your womb doesn't grow, and there is no blood building up inside your uterus. Not having your period in this scenario is safe. If you ever felt something different like symptoms of pregnancy such as sore breasts, check with your doctor or clinician or do a pregnancy test to make sure that everything is okay.

Other benefits that women enjoy with use of the shot include: return to fertility usually within three to nine months, is effective even if someone is overweight, fewer sickle cell crises in women with sickle cell disease, less pain from endometriosis, and decreased risk of endometrial and ovarian cancer. In addition, research supports that Depo can be given right after delivery of a baby and not have a negative effect on either breast milk supply or the baby's development.

In addition to the abnormal bleeding and weight gain as side effects, people taking the shot have also reported depression and other mood changes, decreased bone density, headaches, decreased libido, and breast discomfort, although those are rare. The one medical condition for which the shot absolutely cannot be used is current or recent (within five years) breast cancer. Also, because of bone mineral density losses that can occur after more than two to four years of Depo use, calcium and vitamin D supplementation is important for these patients, as well as discussing alternative short-term options for birth control after four years of use if that is a concern for some patients. However, several studies have shown that bone density loss is reversed back to normal baseline after Depo injections are stopped for one year, and several professional organizations don't place any restrictions on how many years Depo-Provera° can be used in women ages eighteen to forty-five-years-old.

CHAPTER 6.

"He said that he can feel my vaginal ring when we're having sex, so I'm not sure if that's the right method for me."

Vaginal Rings and Patches

FAST FACTS:

- If the vaginal ring bothers you or your partner during sex, you can actually remove it for up to three hours and replace it after you're done having sex. It will still prevent pregnancy as long as you replace it by the third hour.

- Try to place your patch on a front part of your body. That way, if it falls off, you'll more easily notice compared to if it was on your lower back.

The vaginal ring is a combined hormonal contraceptive and contains both estrogen and progestin. It is used by an estimated 1.9 million or 2.6 percent of US women who report using any contraceptive method. The NuvaRing® is 93 percent effective in preventing pregnancy, which means that of 100 women using the ring, about seven will have an unintended pregnancy with typical use. Women who use the vaginal ring (NuvaRing®) insert it vaginally every twenty-eight days or once per month. The FDA approval states that it should be kept in place for twenty-one days and then removed for seven days, during which time a woman will have her monthly menses. However, several studies have shown that the vaginal ring, like other combined hormonal contraceptives, can be used in extended cycles, especially in women who prefer to skip a period. For example, this technique is used commonly when patients ask for options to plan for no menses during a wedding, honeymoon, vacation, or other special event for which having an active flow would be inconvenient. Studies have shown that among thousands of women, the extended use process is safe.

The vaginal ring works by suppressing ovulation; no eggs are released from the ovaries when it is used correctly. Women who use the ring enjoy that it is easy to insert, easy to remove, and comfortable to use, sometimes with a little lubricant placed on the device to ease the insertion process. Sometimes women who are uncomfortable inserting their fingers into their vaginas or who do not use tampons during their menses are reluctant to try the vaginal ring. If my patients are willing to try, we spend time in the office or during a telehealth visit reviewing how to bend the ring between their forefinger and thumb and place it high into the posterior area of the vagina. For women who are cycling and using tampons, the ring can be either left in place if already there or placed into the vagina if the tampon is already there. There is no increased chance of infection as long as the tampons are placed every few hours as appropriate based on package information for different types of tampons.

There are several benefits to the vaginal ring. By the hormones being released vaginally, there are less hormones that make it into the body system, so women usually have less hormonal side effects. When a woman starts using the vaginal ring, pregnancy prevention hormone levels are reached within the first day of use, so back-up with a condom may only be needed for the first twenty-four hours after placement. When you decide to have the ring removed, fertility usually returns within three months. For persons concerned about weight gain, I have great news! Those on the ring do not typically gain weight which is another reason for its popularity among some women.

If your NuvaRing® is coming to you from a mail pharmacy, it will likely arrive in a cooling package, which tries to keep the temperature at or below seventy-seven degrees for optimal stability of the ring device. However, if the temperature has adjusted some by the time it reaches you, it should still be safe to use. The NuvaRing® can be stored at seventy-seven degrees Fahrenheit or room temperature for up to four months. It is important to avoid temperatures above eighty-six degrees and direct sunlight, as higher temperatures can cause the medicines in the ring to break down and not be as effective for pregnancy prevention. A newly FDA-approved vaginal ring (Annovera®) offers one full year of pregnancy prevention, and it does not have to be refrigerated when not in use. It can be left in place for twenty-one days and removed for seven days, cleaned appropriately, and then placed back into the vagina for twenty-one more days.

There are sometimes scenarios in which women forget to take the NuvaRing® out or they realize that it has fallen out. In those situations, if you are less than forty-eight hours late with inserting a new NuvaRing® and you've had sex, insert the new NuvaRing* as soon as you realize it and keep the ring in until your regularly scheduled ring removal day. If you are more than forty-eight hours late with inserting a new ring, in addition to the two steps above, use a back-up method like condoms or avoid sex until you've had the new ring in place for seven consecutive days.

The patch, also known as OrthoEvra*, (Xulane* is the generic version) is a thin, beige plastic device that looks like a square bandage; it is a well-designed combination contraceptive method that delivers medicine through the skin. The patch works by blocking the ovaries from releasing eggs and by thickening the cervical mucous to keep sperm out. The effectiveness of the patch to prevent pregnancy takes one week after you start using it to be fully effective so a back-up method like a condom is required during that time. The patch is not recommended for women with BMI > 30 as it has not been shown to be as effective in preventing pregnancy for women in this weight group.

Women who use this form of birth control enjoy the flexibility of a weekly application. A new patch is applied to the lower abdomen, upper torso, buttocks, or upper arm once per week and provides seven days of birth control protection. Users of this form of birth control apply a new seven-day patch every week for three weeks, and then on week four, no patch is applied, and menses occur during this fourth week. When applying the patch, be sure to clean and dry the part of the body where it will be applied. During the course of the week, if you notice that the patch is no longer on the area where you applied it, call your doctor to see what next steps might be best based on where you are in your four-week cycle.

Although the patch has been available since 2002, after reports of twice the risk of blood clots compared with the pill, fewer women chose the patch for their contraception. For both the patch and the ring, women who are thirty-five or older, who smoke cigarettes, who have ever had blood clots in their legs, arms, lungs, or eyes, who have a familial disorder that makes your blood clot faster than normal, or who have ever had a stroke or a heart attack, should not use the vaginal ring or the patch. Breast cancer and uterine cancer are also contraindications for these methods, but there are many options that don't include estrogen or that have no hormones at all that can be considered for highly effective pregnancy prevention for women who may be in these high-risk groups.

CHAPTER 7.

"I'm done, yo! I want my tubes tied, cut, burned, and thrown away!"

Permanent Sterilization

FAST FACTS:

- Getting your fallopian tubes tied should be considered permanent sterilization. If you're not sure, consider long-term reversible contraception instead.

- There are various surgical options when fallopian tubes are being tied.

- For male partners, getting their tubes tied is the equivalent of a vasectomy and is also permanent sterilization.

This is a frequent topic of conversation with my patients. "What happens when someone gets their tubes tied, and can they be untied later?" Tubal ligations or disrupting the fallopian tubes as the pathway to fertilization can be done in a variety of ways; my preference is to tie, cut, and/or burn. Other clinicians might place a small clamp on each tube; that crushing effect on the tube causes them to be blocked. No matter which method is used, tubal ligations are considered permanent sterilization and should NOT be considered reversible. Many women who initiate the tubal ligation discussion are DONE with childbearing and are eager to hear more details and sign the consent form. However, if a woman is not certain that she has completed childbearing, then discussing a LARC may be more appropriate and can provide her protection for as long as ten to twelve years.

Tubal ligations are the most popular form of birth control for women in the thirties to forties age group because many women in this age range have decided that they are done with their childbearing. However, when women in their twenties have this procedure, they are more likely to have regrets in later years, especially if they meet a new partner who does not already have children of their own. It is also the case that many OB/GYNs don't feel comfortable doing tubal ligations for patients who are twenty-five or younger. While reproductive autonomy must be respected, ensuring women have all the information they need is a vital part of the decision process. If there's any chance they might change their minds in the future, reversing a tubal ligation (putting the tubes back together through surgery) is not an easy thing to do, depending on a woman's insurance coverage and other anatomic factors. If not covered by insurance, the surgical procedure to reverse a tubal ligation is at least $20,000, much more expensive than using a LARC until you are 100 percent sure about not having any more children. The other option after a tubal ligation could be assisted reproductive technology, such as in vitro fertilization or IVF, which is also very costly, and successful pregnancy results aren't guaranteed.

Another option to consider is a vasectomy, whereby the man's "tubes are tied." The male equivalent to a woman's fallopian tubes are the vas deferens. For heterosexual, monogamous couples who have decided to not have any more children or for any man who decides that he does not want to father any more children, a vasectomy is a very safe and effective surgery for contraception. In fact, the first-year typical failure rate for a vasectomy is 0.15 percent, which is even less than the 0.5 percent failure rate for a tubal ligation in someone with fallopian tubes. During a vasectomy, the vas deferens (man's tubes) are cut and tied or sealed to prevent sperm from traveling to the urethra. If sperm cannot enter the urethra, then the semen that is ejaculated has no sperm to travel to fertilize an egg during sex with a woman. Appendix 2 includes a sketch of permanent sterilization techniques for both a fallopian tube and a vas deferens procedure, so that you can see which parts of the reproductive anatomy are involved with these surgical procedures.

Many years ago, male partners of my patients would often universally shut down any discussions about a vasectomy option; vasectomies were very unpopular because many men feared being "cut down there." Also, there was a popular myth that men would never be able to be erect or ejaculate after having a vasectomy; that is not true! Vasectomies are increasingly being considered by men these days for several reasons, including that it is now better understood that men have erections and ejaculate just fine after uncomplicated vasectomies. Also, more people are understanding that vasectomies are more effective in preventing pregnancies than tubal surgery. Also, for women who choose to not have tubal ligations and who may have health issues with hormonal contraception, many male partners are offering to take up that part of the family planning burden. Kudos to them! Vasectomies are a faster procedure with faster recovery times, cheaper in terms of health costs, and are sometimes able to be reversed more easily (compared with tubal ligation) if there's ever a change of heart regarding the ability to have a child in the future. Still, like a tubal ligation, vasectomies should be considered permanent sterilization and only undertaken if future fertility is not desired.

Importantly, there is a window right after the vasectomy procedure during which pregnancy is still possible. To be considered successful, several ejaculations must occur so that all sperm can be cleared from the reproductive tract. The physician must confirm that rare, non-motile sperm only remain in the man's reproductive system, then the surgery can be considered successful. So, for those of you reading this book, please consider this option more seriously, especially if in a partnership where there is certainty about not desiring future children. Permanent sterilization, whether done with the fallopian tubes or the vas deferens, provides most people who absolutely don't want any more children a peace of mind when it comes to worry-free sex. When you add in condoms to prevent any sexually transmitted infections (STIs), including HIV, then for many who may not be in a monogamous partnership, this is the ultimate worry-free sex.

It's also important to note the history of tubal ligations in the US, in which many Black women, Latinas, and Native American women were unethically and unlawfully subjected to forced sterilization (eugenics) during the 1960s-1970s. Some reports of eugenics even extend into the early 2000s and possibly even in 2020 in Georgia, the southeastern US, where reports indicated that hysterectomies were unlawfully done on detained Spanish-speaking women. It is this history that contributes to the requirement for a thirty-day window after a woman with public insurance signs the consent form to have her tubes tied. The thought is that there is less likely to be coercion involved if she has not only had discussions about risks, benefits, and alternatives with her care team but also had at least thirty days to consider her decision and change her mind. Indeed, I've encountered many women who change their minds when asked right before performing the procedure whether they wish to proceed. It is not required for them to share why they have changed their minds; that is always one's prerogative as a patient. In these circumstances, many of my patients will opt for an alternative long-acting contraceptive, which in most cases can be even more effective than permanent sterilization when inserted correctly.

CHAPTER 8.

"Those condoms aren't the right size, and they take away that good-good feeling."

Condoms for Penises, Vaginas, and Anuses (Male and Female Condoms)

FAST FACTS:

- Most male condom sizes are very similar, at least seven inches long (nine inches for those marketed as XXL, Mega, Huge, or Anaconda); most have a similar width (approximately two inches).

- If a male condom doesn't feel right when on an erect penis, explore other sizes until you get the right fit. Too large or too small can lead to other challenges.

- Latex condoms, and likely most polyurethane condoms (for those with latex allergies), protect against most sexually transmitted infections, including HIV infection. However, natural lambskin condoms are not effective protection against STIs or HIV.

Condoms have the dual benefit of decreasing risks of unplanned pregnancies and sexually transmitted infections. Because they are easily accessed and available at most stores, they are very commonly used for contraception. In 2019, an estimated 6.1 million women age fifteen to forty-nine years reported using a male condom during a recent sexual encounter. By covering the tip and shaft of the penis, the male condom serves as a physical barrier and prevents pregnancy by blocking semen from entering the vagina. Male condoms are about 82 percent effective in preventing an unintended pregnancy, which means that eighteen women of 100 who use only male condoms during sex will get pregnant. Female condoms, which are inserted into the vaginal canal during sex, are about 79 percent effective in preventing pregnancy, so slightly less effective than the male condom. Male condoms also prevent most STIs from moving from the penis to the vagina or anus. The better a male condom fits, the more likely it will allow you to have that "good-good feeling."

Condom use increased steadily during the late 1980s-2000s, mostly in response to the newly evolving HIV epidemic and ongoing STI challenges in many communities but in recent years has plateaued and even decreased, especially among high school students who are newer in their sexual experiences. My advice is if you are even thinking about sex with a non-monogamous partner, always keep your own set of condoms with you. If you're in a hot and heavy moment and the other person doesn't have a condom readily available, having one (or several) allows you to continue to enjoy your sex experience uninterrupted.

Male condoms are used much more frequently than female condoms; many people describe female condoms as uncomfortable to navigate as they can be associated with more slippage. Male condoms come in a wide variety of shapes, sizes, flavors, and thicknesses. Many of them have different lubricants, spermicides, and tip shapes, including reservoir tips to hold semen that is ejaculated during sexual orgasm.

Internal condoms have also been known as "female condoms" and can go into a vagina or anus before sex. Internal condoms are made of soft plastic, either polyurethane or nitrile, in the form of a tube that has a closed end. Each end has a ring/rim that helps to create a barrier of protection around either the vagina or anus, depending on how it is used. The closed end ring is inserted deep into either the vagina or anus. If inserted into the vagina, the closed, ring side must cover the cervix, so that sperm does not enter the cervix to fertilize an egg. The safest way to remove this condom is to squeeze the outer ring to keep the semen inside the pouch and gently pull it out of the vaginal canal. Many women like the fact that internal condoms can be placed into the vagina up to eight hours before sex. If a woman is on her cycle and has a tampon in place, the tampon must be removed before inserting the female condom into the vagina. When used in the vagina, the internal condom is about 75-82 percent effective in preventing pregnancy with normal use; effectiveness jumps up to 95 percent when used perfectly each time. While these internal condoms also protect against STIs and HIV, they often don't work as well against STIs compared with condoms that cover the penis (male condoms), likely because they have a looser fit within the vagina.

When it comes to STIs, latex condoms are a great addition to your sexual encounter no matter what type of contraception you choose. While condoms aren't 100 percent effective against all STIs, they do decrease the chance of sexual transmission of gonorrhea, chlamydia, syphilis, trichomoniasis, and HIV. Other STIs, like herpes and human papillomavirus (HPV), aren't 100 percent protected against even with a condom in place because they are viruses that can often be present in the skin areas around the vagina and anus, even if dormant. Many persons who have a positive blood test for the type of herpes that can cause genital lesions report that they never had an outbreak in their genital area. However, someone who has never had a herpes outbreak can still potentially transmit herpes to a partner during sex. Herpes can be complicated in how it behaves, so if you have ever tested positive for herpes, be sure to talk with your clinician about specifics, so that you feel prepared not just for yourself but in case your sex partner(s) has questions. A good online resource for information about herpes is www.asha.org.

Another development in HIV prevention that is helpful when someone is also using condoms and possibly concerned about STI/HIV exposure is pre-exposure prophylaxis or PrEP. Although PrEP is mostly prescribed for and used by gay or same-gender loving men (because of the epidemiology of them being most affected by the US epidemic), it's likely underutilized among women who may be at risk of HIV exposure during unprotected sex. When data are viewed for people in the US, men who have sex with men account for the most new diagnoses of HIV infection, especially men of color who have sex with men. The next groups that are most affected are Black and Hispanic women/Latinas. Regardless of race or ethnicity, there are nationally published PrEP indications for use, and still many physicians and nurse practitioners don't prescribe it enough, often because they haven't obtained a sexual history to fully understand whether a conversation about PrEP would be important to have with patients. So, it's important to know that PrEP is available in the medical world and to advocate for yourself if you meet any of the following indications for PrEP use among sexually-active adults and adolescents: anal or vaginal sex in the past six months, an HIV-positive sex partner (especially if partner has unknown or detectable viral load), or recent bacterial STI (chlamydia, gonorrhea, syphilis), or a history of inconsistent or no condom use with sex partners. Many people don't necessarily have these details about a sex partner and may still be interested in PrEP. For those persons, you must have the following: a documented negative HIV test result before receiving a PrEP prescription, no signs/symptoms of acute HIV infection, normal kidney function, and no contraindicated medicines that won't work with PrEP medicine on board. As of this writing, PrEP is available as pills taken by mouth every day, but new data show that long-acting injectable PrEP looks promising and may be available within the next one to two years.

As you consider your sexual health options with or without condoms, it's important to keep in mind that the cases of STIs in the US have gone up consistently each year for the past five years based on national data from the Centers for Disease Control and Prevention (CDC). Based on the most recent surveillance report from CDC, chlamydia, gonorrhea, infectious syphilis, and congenital syphilis (when a pregnant woman gives birth to a baby with syphilis) have all increased among women and men over the past five years. Congenital syphilis is especially challenging because it points to a likely gap in women getting prenatal care and/or inadequate syphilis screening for pregnant women in prenatal care. For women who receive early and adequate prenatal care, syphilis screening should take place at the first prenatal visit, the third trimester, or about twenty-eight weeks gestation (if they live in a high prevalence community), and when she is admitted to the hospital at the time of delivery. So, as you consider your birth control options, including a condom regardless of which other method you choose is a great way to make sure that you are protected from both an unintended pregnancy and an unwanted STI/HIV. While many STIs can be cured with antibiotic treatments, certain ones like herpes and HIV are viral in nature and can be treated to reduce symptoms and infectivity but not fully cured.

CHAPTER 9.

*"He always pulls out and doesn't come inside me.
That's been working for us."*

Withdrawal, Rhythm Methods, and Other Natural Mechanisms for Birth Control

FAST FACTS:

- It is possible to get pregnant from the pre-ejaculate that is released from the penis during withdrawal from the vagina.

- Many people use the withdrawal method, especially teenagers and young adults.

- Withdrawal does not protect against sexually transmitted infections, including herpes, HPV, or HIV.

- If you have that next-level of self control, the rhythm method and/or withdrawal may be great for you!

Withdrawal or pulling out or "coitus interruptus" happens when a man pulls the penis out of the vagina and away from her genitalia before he ejaculates. Although many sex partners will describe using this method, it is compromised by the fact that sperm-containing semen is often present in pre-ejaculate, and it is possible for a pregnancy to occur if that pre-ejaculate meets up with and fertilizes an egg. In addition, a huge amount of self-control and precise timing are needed from both partners if a man is to successfully pull his penis out in time! I say both partners because withdrawing during this moment can be a challenge for both the male and female partner; that moment is often at the peak of sexual ecstasy. Kudos to those with that level of self-control! Due to these factors, it is estimated that withdrawal is about 75-80 percent effective for preventing pregnancy. And importantly, withdrawal of the penis does not protect against STIs or HIV because while the penis is in the vagina, it has no covering on it and any direct contact of mucous membranes can lead to transmission and/or acquisition of STIs/HIV.

The rhythm method is a form of birth control that uses natural family planning techniques. When a woman gets her period very regularly, the same time every month, she's able to predict when she will ovulate and likely conceive. By counting the days when she will ovulate and possibly conceive, she can then plan which days she needs to avoid sex, or she can decide to use a condom or diaphragm or vaginal gel during just the fertile days of that month. On average, an egg is released from an ovary about 14 ± 2 days after the start of a menstrual cycle. To count correctly, it's important to know that the egg lives for about three to four days (six to twenty-four hours after ovulation), and sperm can live for forty-eight to seventy-two hours or sometimes longer in estrogen-rich cervical mucous. This type of fertility awareness method can be up to 98 percent effective in preventing pregnancy. However, because of the high level of continuous monitoring and self-control required, this method is also often used by couples who are trying to become pregnant, whereby they try to time sexual intercourse based on when ovulation is likely to have occurred.

So, let's talk more about ovulation because certainly ovulation kits have become very popular among women and/or couples trying to plan for their most fertile moments with the goal of having sex, so they can conceive a child. These ovulation kits are used to predict ovulation. They work by a woman checking her urine for luteinizing hormone (LH). LH promotes maturation of an egg in the ovary. LH levels typically increase twenty to forty-eight hours before ovulation, which is called the LH surge. This LH surge can be measured in a woman's urine eight to twelve hours after the LH surge. For women who are using the ovulation kits, they plan for sex or insemination during the two days before ovulation, the day of ovulation, and the day after ovulation, although the best chance of a pregnancy is within twenty-four hours of the LH surge.

For many women who might be breastfeeding, lactational infertility is a "natural method of birth control" and refers to the idea that a woman cannot become pregnant while she is breastfeeding. But I don't want you to get too comfortable with this notion because it is not 100 percent the case at all. It is true that most women who are exclusively breastfeeding the baby will have a delay in return of ovulation after delivering, but some breastfeeding women might ovulate and not realize that they are fertile even before their period returns. Exclusive breastfeeding means that a woman is not giving her baby any supplemental formula and that only her breastmilk is supplying the baby's nutritional needs. To quantify, exclusive breastfeeding means that a baby is being fed at least every four hours during the day and every six hours at night. If you are doing that, this lactational absence of a menstrual cycle can last until your baby is about six months old. After that, many babies are starting to eat other, more solid food, sleep more through the night, and this is when a woman's period will likely return. By six months postpartum, if a woman wishes to prevent or delay a new pregnancy, she should consider adding a different birth control method.

Several birth control options are safe to use while breast-feeding. Some can be started right after you deliver your baby. They include: the shot or Depo-Provera˚, Norplant˚, Skyla˚ and Mirena˚ IUDs, and progestin-only birth control pills. For the first three weeks after delivery because of the increased risk of blood clots and harmful outcomes for a new mom, we don't use any birth control methods that contain the hormone estrogen; these include any combination pills (Appendix 2), the patch, or NuvaRing˚.

Lastly, I want to just briefly mention abstinence, which is 100 percent effective at preventing pregnancy if there is no penile-vaginal intercourse. Sometimes, I'll have patients who believe that if they've had only oral sex anal sex or even just penile-vaginal sex with withdrawal, they are still virgins and practicing abstinence. That is not correct. Oral and anal sex are also forms of sexual intercourse. Penile-vaginal sex even with withdrawal is still sexual intercourse. When you speak with your doctor about sex, remember to be as specific as possible, so that we can offer the best feedback and recommendations based on the types of sex you are having.

CHAPTER 10.

"Doc, call me back, please! The condom broke! Again!"

Emergency Contraception

FAST FACTS:

- Emergency contraception works best if used within five days of unprotected penile-vaginal sex, so never hesitate to call and ask for help if something unexpected happens.

- Although an emergency contraception pill, Plan B, is available over-the-counter in the US, many women still report challenges with obtaining the medicine without a prescription, especially if the pharmacist is not friendly.

- A copper IUD placed within five to ten days after unprotected intercourse reduces the chance of pregnancy by > 99 percent.

Emergency contraception (EC) includes medicines and devices that can be used after intercourse to prevent pregnancy. In clinical medicine, emergency contraception has been long used in cases of sexual assault with women to help prevent an unwanted pregnancy. Since 1998, there have been Food and Drug Administration (FDA)-approved emergency contraception items that are dedicated specifically for that use, compared with before that when clinicians working with sexual assault victims would use higher quantities of birth control pills to achieve the same effect of stopping an egg from being released from the ovaries. Other types of emergencies in which EC might be warranted include a condom breaking or slipping off during sex, missing two or more birth control pills during a monthly cycle, or perhaps recognizing that a vaginal ring or patch is no longer where it's supposed to be.

Importantly, EC does not work when a pregnancy has already implanted into a uterus; it is not an abortion pill. Some people who oppose the use of EC in these emergency situations incorrectly believe that EC is the same as the abortion pill. An abortion pill can be used in circumstances when a woman is early in a pregnancy, up to eleven weeks pregnant (seventy-seven days after the first day of your last period), but it is most effective in stopping a pregnancy when it is used early, like eight weeks or less in their pregnancy. Many women do not realize that they are pregnant until about six weeks, so being able to access care quickly for an undesired pregnancy makes a difference in the types of treatments and the safety of those treatments for women.

The two designated categories of EC are either pills or the copper IUD. EC pills include progestin-only pills that can be purchased over the counter by those who are age seventeen years and older; they are Plan B˚ (Generic versions include: Preventeza˚, Take Action˚, Next Choice One Dose˚, AfterPill˚, and My Way˚). Although no prescription is required for these pills, some women still face challenges when trying to acquire them. Some pharmacies place the pills in locked areas that require asking a sales associate. If you are an already nervous and scared adolescent, this additional barrier could be harm-ful, and in fact, several of my patients have described this as a barrier. Obtaining emergency contraception is often some-thing that many women feel self-conscious about, sometimes even more for older or mature women who feel they might be judged as "they should have known better" or "she's just too grown for that." Ideally, emergency contraception pills should be available, so that persons who need it during an emergency can access them quickly and without judgment, thereby de-creasing the risk of having an unplanned or undesired preg-nancy due to unnecessary barriers.

There is also an EC pill that is only available by prescrip-tion called Ella˚. Ella˚ is a non-hormonal pill which contains ulipristal; ulipristal is a drug that blocks the effects of hor-mones necessary for conception. Ella˚ is even more effective than Plan B˚. When used for up to 120 hours after unprotect-ed sex, the pregnancy rate was only 2 percent, so Ella˚ is 98 percent effective at preventing pregnancy. Women who take Ella˚ must wait at least five days before resuming or starting hormonal birth control. If sexual intercourse happens before a woman sees her next period after taking Ella˚, she should consider using a back-up barrier method like a condom to decrease the chance of an unintended pregnancy.

The other category of EC is the copper IUD. When used in this way, the copper IUD is extremely effective (99 percent of unintended pregnancies prevented). In fact, it is the most effective form of emergency birth control. It must be inserted by your doctor up to five days after you've had unprotected sex, and for those who wish to maintain it as a long-acting form of birth control, it can remain in place for ten to twelve years. That's a win-win situation for someone who may be in a situation desiring both EC and long-term contraception.

The side effects from emergency contraception are not usually serious; they can include headaches, lower abdominal pain or cramps, fatigue, dizziness, nausea, and breast tenderness. Most women describe their symptoms as mild if they have them at all. Women may notice that their period may come a little early or a little late, and spotting is likely in between periods. If you have taken EC and do not get your period more than one week after expected, take a pregnancy test or go to see your doctor. Sometimes a visit to the doctor is necessary because pregnancy hormones called beta-HCG might still be in your system from a previous pregnancy, and special blood tests may be needed to figure out the current status of successful EC versus new pregnancy.

CHAPTER 11.

"It's all about access . . . Can't I borrow birth control from a friend in a pinch?"

Maintaining Access to Birth Control Services and a Healthy Sex Life During a Public Health Emergency

FAST FACTS:

- Like an emergency fund, try to have a six-month supply of your chosen birth control method at home with you, whether it's the pill, the vaginal ring, patch, Depo, or condoms.

- If you can't access your usual provider, consider one of the online platforms for birth control. They can provide most forms of the birth control pill after obtaining a satisfactory medical history from you.

- Become comfortable with self-pleasure, especially if you have a partner who is potentially exposed to a contagious agent when they are working outside of the home during a pandemic.

Girl, no, you cannot borrow birth control from a friend! It's important that you have your own birth control, so that both you and your friend have the contraception that you both need, especially in an emergency when you both might be having more sex than usual. Recent public health emergency events, especially during the COVID-19 pandemic, have underscored the importance of being able to access medications and other prescribed contraceptive methods outside of traditional processes. During the recent COVID-19 emergency, several patients had trouble accessing their birth control (the pill and/or Depo) due to closed pharmacies, pharmacies promising to mail prescriptions and having mailing delays due to both shipments and mail services, and even closed medical offices, so that Depo-Provera shots could not be administered on time within the twelve to thirteen week window.

Pharmacies releasing birth control to women only one month at a time has been a long-term challenge for many women who use the pill and who have Medicaid as insurance. Even though I write prescriptions for a patient to get six months of pill packs at one time, pharmacies won't dispense them that way, often due to insurance barriers. That is unacceptable, and as we saw during the recent public health emergency, many women were caught between a rock and a hard place with likely increased sex at home with their quarantined partners and decreased access to the birth control that they needed to prevent an undesired pregnancy. These scenarios did not allow for much worry-free and joyful sex.

For Depo-Provera*, we learned that many women who were not comfortable giving themselves a deep muscle injection for this method were willing to try the Depo-subQ version of the medicine. Depo-subQ is more of a superficial injection (shorter needle) very much like when someone takes insulin for diabetes treatment. When pharmacies did re-open, many women who were still weary about going to their doctors' offices were open to trying the subQ injection as a compromise which still allowed them to access the birth control method that they had already gotten used to and wished to continue. Depo-SubQ also has approximately 30 percent less hormone, so you may also have less side effects if you use this method.

It's also important to consider online or telehealth options for birth control services. Over the past eight years, there have been a growing number of online and/or app-based telehealth companies that have been offering family planning services after initial online consultations to screen for any serious health concerns. These companies expanded in their reach during the recent public health emergency with COVID-19 and became a go-to resource for thousands of women who needed to continue to access their birth control. Because most contraceptive visits don't require a physical exam, telehealth lends itself to this approach by providing a direct format for counseling regarding contraceptive options and then either mailing the mutually decided upon birth control or sending a prescription to a local pharmacy near the patient. Here is a list of some online companies that provide online prescriptions for hormonal contraception; they vary by states in which services are available, age range for services, and price of birth control:

- Pandia Health (www.pandiahealth.com); this one accepts Medicaid in CA.
- Nurx (www.nurx.com)
- SimpleHealth (www.simplehealth.com)

- Lemonaid Health (www.lemonaidhealth.com)
- HelloAlpha (www.helloalpha.com)
- Maven Clinic (www.mavenclinic.com)
- HealthPartners (www.healthpartners.com)
- Project Ruby (www.prjktruby.com/)
- The Pill Club (www.thepillclub.com)
- Virtuwell (www.virtuwell.com)
- HeyDoctor (www.heydoctor.com)
- PlushCare (www.plushcare.com)
- Planned Parenthood Direct (hwww.plannedparent-hood.org/get-care/get-care-online)

For a full list of online providers that is regularly updated due to the rapid growth of these types of services, please go to: https://freethepill.org/online-pill-prescribing-resources/. This resource includes information about age and state limitations, fees, and whether any insurances are accepted for the various online options.

One thing that has been discussed in scientific and political circles but has not yet come to fruition is the notion of making birth control pills available over-the-counter for women to be able to access and purchase them when needed, especially during emergencies like the COVID-19 pandemic. Can you imagine the thousands of women who would have been able to prevent a lapse in their pill use if they were able to access what they needed over-the-counter? Although over 100 countries around the globe allow sale of the pill over-the-counter (and data show it to be safe), this has not been approved for the US. Despite data showing safety, we have a long way to go to get there in this country, and while I'm hopeful, there may be new federal legal challenges to these efforts that could slow down discussions that have been taking place.

Another option to consider getting what you need is a concierge medicine practice. Concierge gynecology practices allow you 24/7 access to your provider and specialized care to coordinate not only delivery of your birth control and other medicinal needs but also a full range of holistic and tailored patient care services through flexible appointment and tele-health options. This approach is especially vital for women who are leading very busy lives and having a hard time ac-cessing what they need in a timely manner. For these patients, appointments are able to occur at a place and time that you choose; your provider often comes directly to you.

As a busy mom and career person working outside of the home, offering this type of service to my patients became very important to me. Too many of us slip through the cracks for ourselves as we're caring for others or doing what we need to do to make ends meet. When I created Control Concierge, my primary concern was "GYN care on your time." Check out www.controlconcierge.com to learn more about how to access this type of concierge GYN care.

Another topic that was raised more often by some of my patients during the pandemic was how to have sex during a whirlwind time of social distancing, possibly having a part-ner who was an essential worker and potentially exposed whenever they went to work, or even wanting to kiss your partner when you are hearing about things being transmitted through respiratory droplets and other close contact. During these times, self-pleasure and mutual masturbation were occurring more frequently, and many folks who were initially uncomfortable found themselves becoming comfortable with these sexual options. If/when similar outbreaks happen in the future, these will continue to be valid and safe approaches to healthy sexuality.

More sex toys were used for self-pleasure during this recent pandemic; it's okay to experiment and enjoy what makes you feel good! Try out new things if you are in a situation where you are not able to access the partnered sexual activity you may have been used to getting regularly. If using sex toys, it's important to clean those with warm, soapy water after each encounter. Also, it is important to know about mutual masturbation. Mutual masturbation is defined as masturbating separately but together; it boosts moods and also provides an option for emotional connection. Some sex partners even tried wearing dental dams during kissing encounters; the challenge with this is that it would not be possible to breathe if both the mouth and nose are covered, and that would be the only way to be protected if you thought someone was either positive for an infectious agent or that they were at risk of being positive. What this pandemic has taught us universally is that we have to think differently about how we prepare for our birth control and sexual pleasure options in the future, so that we are not caught off-guard when the desire hits us!

CHAPTER 12.

"I'm on the thick side, and my blood pressure has been up.
Can I still use my pill?"

Considerations When You Have
Other Medical Diagnoses

FAST FACTS:

- If you have high blood pressure, there are safer options than the combination birth control pill; let's consider one of the other options.

- Some birth control options haven't been studied in women at certain weights, or we find that some medicines that prevent pregnancy are less effective above a certain weight. That is why we sometimes consider weight when you are deciding between your options.

- No matter what your medical situation is, there is a safe and effective birth control option for you if you feel you need one.

Many people in the US are also managing medical diagnoses as they try to navigate their sex lives and use of birth control. For any medical diagnosis, it is vital that you share as much as you can with your healthcare provider, so that they can give you the best possible guidance and recommend methods that are safest for you based on your pregnancy prevention goals.

In this chapter, we'll discuss some of the most common medical diagnoses that we see in clinical practice, including obesity, lupus, chronic hypertension, and sickle cell disease.

Obesity is defined as a BMI of thirty and above, and obesity is increasing in most states in the US. Overweight is a BMI of twenty-five to twenty-nine. When my patients describe themselves as thick or big-boned, this doesn't necessarily mean they are obese; that may just be how they describe themselves. When we calculate BMIs, we measure someone's weight (in kilograms) divided by the square of his or her height (in meters). For combined hormonal contraceptives, including the pill, patch, and vaginal ring, there's an increased risk of venous thromboembolism (VTE) or a blood clot inside their vein that can move to another place in their body for women with BMIs > 35. However, data show that the pregnancy prevention benefit of these methods are not diminished among women with higher BMIs. Still, it's important to be optimally safe while trying to prevent pregnancy.

For women with diabetes mellitus, the ideal situation for birth control means having well- controlled blood sugar. If that's in place, then most forms of birth control that are safe for women without diabetes are also safe for women with diabetes. Most providers will start with a low-dose birth control pill for these patients, but the vaginal ring, LARCs, and barrier methods also work well in women with diabetes. If a woman does start a new pill and notices shifts in her sugar levels when she does finger sticks, trying an alternative birth control pill may be appropriate unless she wants to try something else altogether.

Hypertension or high blood pressure may be a contraindication for combined hormonal contraceptives depending on how well controlled the blood pressure is. For example, if your blood pressure is above 160/100 even with medication, birth control pills that contain estrogen (combination pills) are not for you. If there are other factors like obesity or smoking of cigarettes, the risk of blood clots and stroke are too high. For these patients, most providers would suggest a progestin-only or a non-hormonal option for birth control. The copper IUD is great in women who may have these risk factors because it has no hormones and is highly effective at preventing pregnancy. The IUD could be removed whenever she decides that she was ready to have another child. There are also some women who after considering the long-term impact of chronic health conditions like high blood pressure may decide to opt for permanent sterilization with a tubal ligation if they no longer wish to have more children.

Smoking cigarettes, especially if age thirty-five years or older, is a strict contraindication for using combination birth control pills and most other hormonal methods due to the increased risk of DVT, myocardial infarctions, and strokes. The safest options for these patients include non-hormonal methods. Many of my patients who are thirty-five and older opt for permanent sterilization if they have completed childbearing.

Lupus is a multi-organ system disease, and how it shows up varies with each patient. Many people with lupus have an increased risk of heart disease and clot formation in their veins and arteries; these contribute to more complications for the mother and fetus during a pregnancy if there is a lupus flare. Because over half of those with lupus are diagnosed between ages sixteen to fifty-five years, reproductive health needs are a vital part of their overall healthcare discussion and plan. Labs that are often checked in patients diagnosed with lupus are: 1) antiphospholipids, and 2) platelets. When antiphospholipids are present or unknown, there is an increased risk for VTE or blood clots with estrogen-containing and progestin-only methods of birth control. However, the copper IUD is very effective when antiphospholipid antibodies are present. If someone has platelets that are very low (< 50,000), use of De-po-Provera or a copper IUD may be risky; patients who select these have to be watched more closely. Alternative options such as barrier methods, lower dose pills, a vaginal ring, or an implant are better options to consider in these cases.

Women who have sickle cell disease (SCD) have to be managed carefully because some studies have shown that maternal mortality rate is more than ten times higher for patients with SCD compared to women without SCD. So, contraceptive counseling is a vital part of GYN care for women with SCD if they are interested in discussing the options available to them for pregnancy timing. Most times, progestin-only contraceptives, especially Depo-Provera, are great options because they have a lower risk of painful sickle cell crises and also a lower level of anemia. There is a concern about combination birth control options causing more blood vessel blockage and therefore more pain; for that reason, many providers will not prescribe these as often so as to not (even if only theoretically) cause more bone or crisis pain.

I often get questions from perimenopausal women who are concerned about not slipping up and having a "change of life baby." Ladies, I understand! ☺ For women in this group who don't smoke, don't have hypertension, history of blood clots, diabetes, or other risk factors, low-dose combination birth control pills are a great option. The pill has many benefits for perimenopausal women including treatment of hot flashes and night sweats, preventing an unintended pregnancy, decreased blood loss during cycles, better cycle control, decreased bone loss, and protection against some gynecologic cancers. Vaginal dryness may also be decreased among perimenopausal women depending on the hormonal combinations in the pill prescribed. Before starting a low-dose pill during perimenopause, it's important to make sure that you are up-to-date with your routine Pap and screening mammogram, if you are in the age range for these recommended screenings.

CHAPTER 13.

"How close are we to a pill for men?
It's their turn for real!"

Birth Control Options for Men

FAST FACTS:

- This is a very short chapter, y'all!

There's just not that much out there for men…yet. Many women ask, appropriately, "What's up with more birth control options besides vasectomy for men?!" It is true that women have carried the birth control burden since the beginning of contraceptive availability. Studies show that about 50 percent of men *say* that they would be willing to share in the responsibility of birth control, so that the burden won't continue to fall solely on the partner with the uterus. In recent years, there's been a pill being studied for men, but it is still in development and being researched to be sure it is safe and efficacious. But what will be the reality of men taking a pill for birth control once it is available and FDA-approved? And how many of us women will fully trust turning this over to our male partners for them to handle?

Another option being considered for men is a contraceptive gel that would have to be used daily. There is an ongoing study in California in which men who volunteer rub the contraceptive gel onto their shoulders. The gel works by blocking natural testosterone production in the testes thereby reducing sperm production. While doing this, the gel is also supposed to have some amount of replacement testosterone to help men keep a normal sex drive. It's estimated that the man's sperm count would be low enough to prevent pregnancy in four to six months. In this study, the man would stop using the gel after twelve months and would continue to be followed for four months until his sperm count returned to normal range. We'll have to see how this works out, but it certainly is an exciting new development in the world of contraception.

Also being discussed for men is a process called reversible inhibition of sperm under guidance (RISUG) in which men receive a substance injected directly into their vas deferens (the tubes that are tied during a vasectomy). The injected substance works by inactivating sperm in the vas deferens, which then prevents the sperm from leaving the male tubes. If the sperm does not leave the vas deferens, it can't make its way to the woman's uterus or fallopian tubes to find an egg. However, RISUG has been in development for many years. One thing that folks debate about all the time is whether women will fully trust a male contraceptive. After all, if a contraceptive fails, it is women who bear the greatest responsibility regarding her pregnancy or abortion options. For these reasons, some women are not 100 percent certain about fully relinquishing control to men. But it's nice to be able to have male-focused options as a future possibility.

CHAPTER 14.

"How much does that cost? I have to make sure
it's in my budget."

The Highs and Lows of Birth Control Access and Costs

FAST FACTS:

- The costs of birth control are immensely affected by what is covered in health insurance plans.

- The Affordable Care Act significantly reduced out-of-pocket birth control costs for women.

- Women without healthcare insurance or access remain at highest risk of unintended pregnancy; free and low-cost birth control options are vital for many women in the US.

Birth control costs can certainly add up over time, which is one reason why costs being covered by the Affordable Care Act was such a helpful thing for so many women who may have had access challenges and cost barriers. Now, even though the ACA continues to face legal challenges, most birth control options except for IUDs depending on your employer can be obtained without co-pays.

The range of birth control costs are as follows (this does not include possible costs of a provider visit):

The Pill: $0-$50 per month, initial physical exam = $20–$200; annual cost = $20–$800

IUD: $0–$1300 up front if not covered by insurance; for annual costs, divide by number of years your IUD is in place.

Condoms: free at some local health clinics or $2.50–$5.00 per condom at drug stores. Costs depend on how often you are sexually active.

Depo-Provera: $30–$75 every three months for the injection; $120–$300 per year and possible additional fee to receive injection at physician's office

NuvaRing: $30–$35 per monthly ring; $360–$420 per year

Patch: $30–$35 per month; $360–$420 per year (same as NuvaRing)

Annovera vaginal ring: $2098 for one ring to be used for one year

Sterilization: $1000 for men and $6,000 for women upfront costs if not covered by insurance

Phexxi: (non-hormonal, vaginal gel) $267.50 for a box of twelve applicators.

It's important to note that even today, especially with ongoing challenges to the contraceptive part of the Affordable Care Act, many groups of women continue to have challenges accessing the birth control that they need. These challenges overlap directly with the reproductive justice framework mentioned in the beginning of this book. Particularly in "contraceptive deserts" (areas where there is less than one health provider or clinic for every 1,000 women) in the US, there are approximately 20 million women who lack access to birth control. Sadly, it is the most vulnerable women in these situations who are unable to access what they need; this includes women in more rural areas, racial/ethnic minority groups of women, and women who may be from migrant populations.

Ideally, we should be able to ensure a full-service health center and/or healthcare provider in every US county. However, we are not there yet. For women who run into these barriers with accessing their birth control due to costs, there is an organization which can provide some help. The National Women's Law Center (www.nwlc.org/coverher) has a program which offers help and guidance to women who have questions or concerns about accessing their birth control. The phone number is: 1-866-745-5487, and the website is www.coverher.org. Since 2012, they've helped several hundred thousand women in the US access the birth control they need. Their motto is: "Access to birth control is essential," and they provide vital services to women to help ensure their control and freedom.

As we consider the groups most affected by birth control access challenges, it is also important to consider that pregnancies, whether planned or not, affect different groups of women differently in this country. For women of color, who are disproportionately affected by contraceptive deserts, this is particularly troubling because they are also most affected by the dismal maternal mortality rates in this country. The maternal mortality rate in the US has doubled between 1986 and 2020; we have the highest maternal mortality rate when compared with other industrialized nations in the world. These disparities are a public health failure that have generated increased attention and policy shifts in recent years, especially because approximately 60 percent of pregnancy-related deaths are preventable. Persistently, women of color have been disproportionately affected by maternal mortality; Black/African American women and American Indian/Alaska Native women are 3.3 and 2.5 times more likely to die from pregnancy-related causes than white women in the US. We have to do better for our women along the entire spectrum of family planning care, and part of doing better is ensuring all have what they need for access to both family planning and prenatal and postpartum care should they choose to have a pregnancy. When/if they make that choice, it should be with a healthcare system that helps ensure that a woman's health and safety both during and up to one year after the pregnancy are considered because pregnancy-related deaths can occur for up to one year after the end of the pregnancy.

There have been some recent policy movements regarding maternal mortality. After several high profile and devastating maternal deaths in the US, H.R. 1318 or the Preventing Maternal Deaths Act was signed into law at the end of 2018. The goal of this law is to "support states in their work to save and sustain the health of mothers during pregnancy, childbirth, and in the postpartum period to eliminate disparities in maternal health outcomes for pregnancy-related and pregnancy-associated deaths, to identify solutions to improve healthcare quality and health outcomes for mothers, and for other purposes" (www.govtrack.us/congress/bills/115/hr1318).

Other maternal health bills have been introduced since this was signed into law, but they have not yet moved forward through the federal process to be made into laws. These initial steps signal that maternal health is being taken increasingly seriously by our country's leaders; that progress, even in 2021, is a good thing.

CHAPTER 15.

"What else is new in birth control? It just seems like timing a pregnancy should be easier to do!"

New Contraceptive Methods for Women

FAST FACTS:

- There are a few new options on the market, and development is ongoing to try to find the next best thing that is effective and easy to use.

- If you really want the cutting-edge, nerdy stuff, go to www.ctiexchange.org and read about what's on the horizon in "Advancing Contraceptive Innovation" in the Calliope (Contraception Pipeline Database) section.

Just approved for use in 2020, Phexxi™ is a newly available, FDA-approved, vaginal, non-hormonal, bio-adhesive gel that can be used for the prevention of pregnancy in females of reproductive age. It is intended as an on-demand method of contraception and can be used right before penile-vaginal sex (up to one hour before); it must be re-applied before each act of sexual intercourse. A prescription is required for this; it is not over-the-counter at this time. By the gel creating an acidic environment in the vagina before intercourse, the more basic sperm become less motile and less likely to pass from the vagina through the cervix to potentially reach an egg. The estimated failure rate is about fifteen out of 100, so it will likely prevent pregnancy about 85 percent of the time. Also, this cannot be used in anyone who has recurrent UTIs and should not be used concurrently with a vaginal ring. The main adverse reactions reported with this include: vulvovaginal burning or itching, urinary tract infections, and sometimes sex partners describe feeling some local discomfort.

A new vaginal ring, Annovera™, was approved by FDA in 2018, so now there are two options for vaginal rings on the market. It has both estrogen and progestin. Unlike the other vaginal ring that has been around for over a decade, this ring can be used for one year or thirteen cycles (in for twenty-one days, out for seven days)! This gives you more control based on fewer pharmacy visits; you just have to keep it clean with mild soap and lukewarm water in-between insertions. With this ring, it is important to avoid oil or silicon-based vaginal products, but water-based lubricants are fine. Also, this new ring does not have any latex in it, so it is also good for latex-sensitive persons.

A new contraceptive patch, Twirla˚, was approved for use in 2020. It has both estrogen and progestin. Like OrthoEvra˚, this patch is changed weekly for a 21/7 day cycle. This patch is contraindicated in persons with a BMI $\geq$ 30 kg/m^2. Like the other patch, this can be applied to the abdomen, buttocks, or upper torso as long as the skin is clean and dry. Twirla˚ is twice the size of the old patch, and it has no latex; it is made from Skinfusion˚, a new, five-layer technology. This Twirla˚ patch can be started within the first twenty-four hours of menses, or else seven days of a back-up method is needed.

A new progestin-only pill was approved in 2019; it is called Slynd™. It is intended for use on a 24/4 day cycle. It may also work for continuous use, but that approach has not been studied yet. This works by suppression of ovulation, so no eggs are released. This has a higher dose of progestin; it can be missed up to twenty-four hours, and no back-up method is needed. Remember that for the other progestin-only MiniPill, a back-up method is needed if you are just three hours late with taking that MiniPill.

The Caya diaphragm is a new hormone-free, contoured diaphragm which prevents sperm from entering the uterus. It should be used with the Caya gel to work most effectively, and it should be inserted into the vagina any time before any sexual encounter. If the diaphragm was inserted > 2 hours before sex or if another sex encounter is happening, more gel must be applied into the vagina on the diaphragm. The Caya diaphragm must be removed by six hours after sex has occurred. The Caya diaphragm is reusable for up to two years before having to replace it with a new diaphragm.

PART III.

YOU ARE IN CONTROL

"If you don't take control over your time and your life, other people will gobble it up. If you don't prioritize yourself, you constantly start falling lower and lower on your list."

—Michelle Obama

CHAPTER 16.
What Does Control Look Like for You?:
Defining Your Sexual Freedom Formula

FAST FACTS:

- Only you can determine what control looks like for you; no one else can do that.

- Your freedom = what fulfills your soul and brings you peace of mind.

- Always remember…your oxygen mask first.

When we are in control, we are often self-aware and fully in touch with our desires for our lives. For women, this is often also affected by what is on our plates and what we feel we must do for others. So many of us are leading very busy, almost overwhelming lives, with many different to-do lists to conquer. Compared with men, more women are nurturers and caregivers who often put others' needs before our own. A vital part of being in control is to ensure that your own needs are met as a priority; those include personal and professional needs and especially self-care needs. You must ensure that you remain high on your list! More and more, we are learning that self-care is a way for us all to become more productive and present persons in various aspects of our lives and to ensure that we don't lose ourselves as we care for others. And self-care doesn't have to mean long vacations or extended time away from others. Self-care can be part of our daily routines, mini-moments that we allow ourselves during the day. Sometimes, for me, it's as simple as taking a walk, sitting still on a bench in the sunshine, lighting a candle, spending quiet time in a bookstore, or listening to a favorite playlist of music. We can have control by being deliberate about prioritizing ourselves and by being more in-tuned with what we need.

Birth control is often part of a woman's lifelong journey toward self-awareness, freedom, and overall control of her choices. Over 99 percent of women have used birth control at some point during their reproductive years in an effort to prevent an unintended pregnancy. Many women will spend about 75 percent of these reproductive years trying to avoid an unwanted or poorly timed pregnancy. So, to get to this chapter which requires some self-reflection, I wanted to make sure that you were aware of and comfortable with the different options available to you just in case birth control at this time or in the near future helps you with your personal goals for control and sexual freedom.

Another aspect of being in control includes our sexuality and having a mindset that is constantly evolving toward freedom. Freedom doesn't mean that you leave a happy, partnered relationship, if you are partnered, rather it means that you are able to be your most free self, whether you are partnered or not. The mindset for controlled, free sexuality includes our surroundings, the sex-related stimulants that are part of our environments. Mindset involves using all of our senses. Which smells, sights, thoughts, tastes, and touches are signals for you to feel most free? Maybe it's a certain candle scent, or an organized home, or partner prepared meal, or the knowledge that you are protected with birth control and not worried about a pregnancy that is not well-timed. Take a moment to think about your sexuality mindset triggers and write them down. For many women, a positive sexuality mindset is also tied to body image, so as we improve our relationship with our bodies, regardless of size or imperfections, our access to sexual pleasure, whether alone or with a partner, improves.

Part of strengthening one's control of one's sexuality is ensuring that women understand and believe several things: 1) Sex is a basic human function, and it affects overall health and happiness, 2) Women need accurate sexual health information, so that they can make the best choices for themselves, including choices regarding sexual desire and when and whether or not they choose to have children, 3) When you have a good foundational relationship with your own sexuality, you are better able to be fully present and mindful for your partner if you choose to have one. For some, that may include pleasuring yourself whether as part of self-care or to share what works for you with a current or future partner, 4) Sex is good for our overall health; it is linked to more happiness, less stress, better memory, and improved moods, 5) When partnered sex is consensual and done with a healthy self-sexuality, it can be an ultimate expression of pleasure, intimacy, and connection.

As you grow on your sexual journey, knowing your own sexual pleasure is a vital part of ensuring that your needs are understood and met. So, as you begin to consider your path to control and freedom, really take some time to sit with yourself and think about what that looks like for you. Take the time to explore your body. What bodily part brings you the most pleasure? Explore it and be comfortable with it. Play with it. That may include toys, and that's great too. Sometimes after a long day, part of your wind-down can include a hot shower or bath, lighting a scented candle, and giving yourself a few moments of self-care. Because our lives are often so busy, many women have to plan this in advance. This may include making arrangements for ensuring that everyone else is out of the house, so that no one comes into your space to disturb you. Try to be creative with it. The main thing is to just plan it or else it will never get done. As children get older, if you have any, and you have fewer balls in the air, it will likely get easier for you to carve out these moments. The more you do these self-care or love yourself moments, the more you will understand how vital they are for your overall well-being.

Another aspect of being in control and reaching maximum freedom is truly understanding what it means to put on your oxygen mask first and then *really* doing it. Love yourself first, then help others. For many of us, this doesn't come naturally, especially women. When I started to put my oxygen mask on first, I started planning me-time as well as son-time. I started planning and participating in girls' trips as well as my annual mom-son adventures. I made sure that I attended and enjoyed those live music concerts that give me so much life. I prioritize solo time as well as time with a partner. When you first start to do it, it won't feel comfortable. People will start to ask you questions, maybe even judge you a little. That's okay. Your control and your freedom are not intended for anyone else to understand, and when you are ultimately free, you will be less and less concerned about what others think. Your joy will be so visible that others will start to ask different questions in an effort to start to tap into their own freedom like yours. It is a joy to help others find their own control and freedom just because they are so moved by watching you on your freedom journey. Embrace that; the more women we bring into this space, the better.

I want you to take some time and be intentional about this next part as you move closer toward worry-free, joyful sex. The sexual freedom formula has five steps:

1. Awareness of self (What does freedom look like to you?)

2. Options (know your options—birth control, safe sex)

3. Acquire (your chosen birth control and/or safe sex method(s), if any)

4. Establish (a safe space for your sexual freedom, whether solo or partnered)

5. Activate (your best life, based on your choices above)

So, what's next for you? Be sure to reflect on what's in this closing chapter and the previous chapters to consider all of your options, whether for birth control or for sexual health and freedom. Make a plan for how you gain or maintain control. Write down what you seek in the coming weeks, months, and years. I've provided some space for your notes on the next page. I've had many patients successfully take this journey and describe the freedom and renewed energy they feel during this process. There is healing in removing shackles, whether real or imagined, and having the life you desire. This journey is an ongoing one, even for me. And the more you plan, the easier it will be to take steps, even small ones toward understanding and embracing what control looks like for you. So, are you ready? Let's get started.

NOTES

NOTES

NOTES

NOTES

NOTES

NOTES

NOTES

NOTES

NOTES

NOTES

AFTERWORD

I'm eternally grateful to all of the women I've encountered on my journey, from family and friends to patients. I've learned something about control and freedom from all of you. By writing this book, I wanted to pay tribute to all of you, and in turn, help the next group of women who may be seeking more control and freedom. So, this is for that busy, overwhelmed woman who has been trying to pull it altogether without letting anything slip through the cracks. I SEE you! I am excited that you are on your own journey for more control and freedom, and I am here to help you if needed. Thank you for all the ways you continue to show up, even as you are on your own journey. Others see you too, and whether they comment on your evolution or not, thank you for being an example for them as well. You are in control!

APPENDIX 1.
Types of Birth Control Pills (1)

Type of pill	Combination (progestin + estrogen)						Progestin-only
	Monophasic	Biphasic	Triphasic	Quadriphasic	Extended cycle	Continuous cycle	Minipill
	(steady dose of hormones through the entire month of pills, except for the inert pills)	(two sets of pills at different strengths until the inert pills)	(three different progestin doses and one dose of estrogen throughout the month, until inert pills)	(four hormone strengths that try to mimic a woman's natural hormone changes during the month)	(deliver monophasic hormones for 91 days so that women only have 4 periods per year)	(continuous days of taking active pills with no breaks at all, so no periods)	(consistent progestin dose throughout the month; no inactive pills and no breaks between packs)
Number of hormone strengths	1	2	3	4	1 or 3	1	1
Menstrual cycle changes	Shorter or lighter periods	No change	Little or no change	Little or no change	4 periods per year	No periods at all	Lighter but longer periods
Likelihood of spotting or breakthrough bleeding	Depends on estrogen dose	Low	Low	High if you miss a dose	High	High	Moderate; high if you miss a dose
Likelihood of other side effects, like acne, weight gain, mood changes	Low	Moderate	High	Low	Low	Low	Low
Examples of pill brand names	Aviane Junel FE 1/20 Apri	Azurette Necon LO Loestrin FE	Ortho Tri-cycen Camrese Tri-previfem	Natazia	Seasonique Jolessa Camreselo	Amethyst	Jolivette Micronor Norethindrone

107

APPENDIX 2.
Sketch of What Is Cut, Tied, or Burned During Permanent Sterilization with a Female or Male

The blue, dashed lines indicate where tubes are either tied, cut or burned during a sterilization procedure.

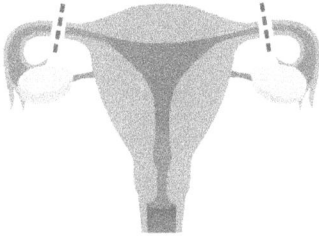

FEMALE STERILIZATION
TUBAL LIGATION

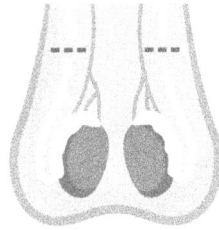

MALE STERILIZATION
VASECTOMY

REFERENCES

1. Hatcher, R. A., A. L. Nelson, J. Trussell, C. Cwiak, P. Cason, M. S. Policar, A. Edelman, A. R. A. Aiken, J. Marrazzo, and D. Kowal, eds. *Contraceptive Technology*. 21st ed. New York, NY: Ayer Company Publishers, Inc., 2018.

2. Ross, L. J., and R. Solinger. *Reproductive Justice: An Introduction*. Oakland, CA: University of California Press, 2017.

3. Sundstrom, S., and C. Delay. *Birth Control: What Everyone Needs to Know*. New York, NY: Oxford University Press, 2020.

4. Franks, A. *Margaret Sanger's Eugenic Legacy: The Control of Female Fertility*. Jefferson, NC: McFarland & Company, Inc., 2005.

ABOUT THE AUTHOR

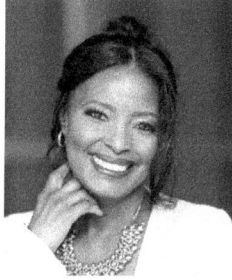

Dr. Madeline Sutton is a board-certified OB/GYN with more than twenty years' experience. She received her BS in Psychology from Georgetown University and her MD and MPH from Columbia University's College of Physicians and Surgeons and Mailman School of Public Health. She previously served on the board of Physicians for Reproductive Health and spent more than two decades as a medical epidemiologist for the Centers for Disease Control and Prevention (CDC).

Along with mentoring early career scientists and medical students, Dr. Sutton participates in medical missions in Haiti and Ghana. She also serves in many community endeavors as an active member of Delta Sigma Theta Sorority, Inc. You can find her book *Our Communities, Our Sexual Health: Awareness and Prevention for African Americans* in a bookstore near you.

Originally from Harlem, New York, Dr. Sutton resides in Stone Mountain, Georgia, with her three sons and black golden doodle.

Learn more at www.InControlBook.com

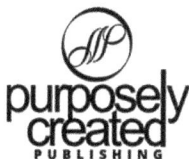

CREATING DISTINCTIVE BOOKS
WITH INTENTIONAL RESULTS

We're a collaborative group of creative masterminds with a mission to produce high-quality books to position you for monumental success in the marketplace.

Our professional team of writers, editors, designers, and marketing strategists work closely together to ensure that every detail of your book is a clear representation of the message in your writing.

Want to know more?
Write to us at info@publishyourgift.com
or call (888) 949-6228

Discover great books, exclusive offers, and more at
www.PublishYourGift.com

Connect with us on social media

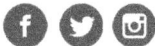

@publishyourgift